The Anti-inflammatory Diet Code

How to Reduce Inflammation

To

Build Immune System Naturally

Dr. Cliff Lawrence

Copyright

TABLE OF CONTENTS

INTRODUCTION

Inflammation is a normal mechanism that your body uses to repair and protect itself.

Inflammation, on the other hand, can be dangerous if it becomes persistent.

Chronic inflammation can persist for weeks, months, or years, and it can cause a variety of health concerns.

Having said that, there are several things you may take to decrease inflammation and enhance your overall health.

This article covers a comprehensive anti-inflammatory food and lifestyle strategy.

What exactly is inflammation?

Inflammation is your body's defense mechanism against infection, disease, or damage.

As part of the inflammatory response, your body produces more white blood cells, immune cells, and anti-infective molecules known as cytokines.
Acute (short-term) inflammation is characterized by redness, discomfort, heat, and swelling.

Chronic (long-term) inflammation, on the other hand, frequently occurs throughout your body without any obvious signs. Diabetes, heart disease, fatty liver disease, and cancer are all caused by this form of inflammation.
Chronic inflammation can also occur when people are overweight or stressed.
When doctors examine for inflammation in your blood, they look for C-reactive protein (CRP), homocysteine, TNF alpha, and IL-6.

IN SUMMARY,

Inflammation is a defense process that helps your body to fight infection, disease, or damage. It can also be chronic, resulting in a variety of disorders.

PART I

What Is the Cause of Inflammation

Consuming a lot of sugar and high-fructose corn syrup is very bad. It has the potential to cause insulin resistance, diabetes, and obesity.

Consuming a lot of refined carbohydrates, such as white bread, may also lead to inflammation, insulin resistance, and obesity, according to scientists.

Furthermore, trans fats in processed and packaged foods have been found to increase inflammation and harm the endothelial cells that line your arteries.

Trans fats are no longer "Generally Recognized as Safe," hence they should be avoided in most meals.

Another likely reason is vegetable oils, which are found in many processed meals. Regular eating may result in an omega-6 to omega-3 fatty acid imbalance, which some experts believe promotes inflammation.

Excessive alcohol and processed meat consumption can also cause inflammation in the body.

Furthermore, an inactive lifestyle that includes a lot of sitting is a significant non-dietary component that might increase inflammation.

IN SUMMARY,

Inflammation is linked to eating unhealthy meals, drinking alcohol or sugary beverages, and receiving little physical activity.

Your Diet's Function

Eat fewer inflammatory meals and more anti-inflammatory foods to minimize inflammation.

Consume complete, nutrient-dense meals strong in antioxidants and avoid overly processed foods heavy in added sugar and fat.

Antioxidants act by lowering free radical levels. These reactive chemicals are produced naturally as part of your metabolism, but if not controlled, they can cause inflammation.

At each meal, your anti-inflammatory diet should include a healthy mix of protein, carbohydrates, and fat. Make sure you're getting enough vitamins, minerals, fiber, and water.

The Mediterranean diet is one anti-inflammatory diet that has been demonstrated to lower inflammatory markers such as CRP and IL-6.

A low-carb diet also decreases inflammation, which is especially beneficial for persons who have obesity or metabolic syndrome.

Furthermore, vegetarian diets have been associated with lower inflammation.

IN SUMMARY,

Choose a nutrient-dense diet that eliminates processed foods and increases your consumption of healthy, anti-inflammatory, antioxidant-rich foods.

Avoidance Foods

Certain foods have been linked to an increased risk of chronic inflammation.

Consider reducing:

• Sugary drinks: Sugar-sweetened beverages and fruit juices

• White bread, white spaghetti, and so on. • Desserts: cookies, candies, cake, and ice cream.

• Processed meats such as hot dogs, bologna, sausages, and so on.

• Processed snack foods such as crackers, chips, and pretzels.

• Processed seed and vegetable oils such as soybean and maize oil

• Alcohol: Abundant alcohol consumption

IN SUMMARY,

Sugary meals and beverages, processed meat, excessive alcohol, and foods heavy in refined carbohydrates and harmful fats should be avoided or limited.

Foods to Consume

5 Anti-Inflammatory Foods You Should Eat

5 Anti-Inflammatory Foods to Eat According to research, some foods can help reduce chronic inflammation. Learn about anti-inflammatory foods by watching this video.

Include plenty of anti-inflammatory items in your diet:

• Vegetables such as broccoli, kale, Brussels sprouts, cabbage, cauliflower, and so on.

• Fruit: Especially deep-colored fruits like blueberries, pomegranates, grapes, and cherries. • High-fat foods: Avocados and olives.

• Fatty fish: salmon, sardines, herring, mackerel, and anchovies • Nuts: almonds and other nuts • Peppers: bell peppers and chili peppers

• Spices such as turmeric, fenugreek, cinnamon, and others.

• Green tea • Red wine: According to research, resveratrol, a molecule found in wine, has anti-inflammatory qualities and may be beneficial to one's health.

IN SUMMARY,

It is ideal to eat a range of nutrient-dense whole foods that can help to minimize inflammation.

PART II

The 8 Best Ketogenic Diet Foods

What foods are permitted on the keto diet? You'll learn about the healthiest foods in this video in 57 seconds.

Sample Menu for One Day

When you have a plan, it is simpler to stick to your diet. Here's a wonderful starting point for you: a day of anti-inflammatory meals:

Breakfast

• 1 cup (225 grams) of cherries

• 1 cup (110 grams) of mushrooms and 1 cup (67 grams) of kale sautéed in olive oil

• Green tea or water

• 1 cup (125 grams) raspberries, topped with plain Greek yogurt and chopped almonds for lunch • Grilled salmon over a bed of mixed greens with olive oil and vinegar

• Water, unsweetened iced tea

Snack

• Guacamole-topped guacamole-topped bell pepper strips

Dinner

• 1 ounce (30 grams) dark chocolate (ideally at least 80% cocoa)

• 5-10 ounces (140-280 ml) red wine

IN SUMMARY, An anti-inflammatory diet plan should be well-balanced, integrating anti-inflammatory items at each meal.

Other Beneficial Advice

Once you've planned your healthy food, make sure to add the following anti-inflammatory lifestyle habits:

• **Supplements**: Certain supplements, such as fish oil and curcumin, have been shown to lower inflammation.

• **Regular exercise**: Regular exercise helps lower inflammatory markers and lower your risk of chronic illness.

• **Sleep**: It is critical to get enough sleep. Researchers discovered that a lack of sleep boosts inflammation.

IN SUMMARY,

You may increase the effectiveness of your anti-inflammatory diet by taking supplements and getting adequate exercise and sleep.

Advantages of a Better Lifestyle

An anti-inflammatory diet, along with exercise and adequate rest, may have several advantages:

• Relief of arthritis, inflammatory bowel disease, lupus, and other autoimmune illnesses symptoms

Obesity, heart disease, diabetes, depression, cancer, and other disorders are all reduced.

• Lower inflammatory indicators in your blood • Improved blood sugar, cholesterol, and triglyceride levels • Increased energy and mood

IN SUMMARY,

Following an anti-inflammatory diet and lifestyle can improve inflammation indicators and lower your risk of numerous illnesses.

It should be noted that chronic inflammation is harmful and can lead to illness.

In many circumstances, your food and lifestyle can cause or aggravate inflammation.

To achieve optimal health and well-being, choose anti-inflammatory foods, lowering your risk of disease and improving your quality of life.

PART III

5 Foods That Inflame the Body

Many diets, particularly those heavy in added sugar, processed carbohydrates, fried foods, alcohol, and high-temperature-cooked meats, can lead to inflammation and chronic illness.

Depending on the circumstances, inflammation can be beneficial or detrimental.

On the one hand, it's your body's natural defense mechanism when you're hurt or unwell.

It can assist your body to protect against sickness and promote recovery.

Chronic, sustained inflammation, on the other hand, has been linked to an increased risk of diseases such as diabetes, heart disease, and obesity.

Surprisingly, the foods you eat can have a significant impact on inflammation in your body.

The following are 5 foods that can cause inflammation:

1. High fructose corn syrup and sugar

The two most common types of added sugar in the Western diet are table sugar (sucrose) and high fructose corn syrup (HFCS).

Sugar contains 50% glucose and 50% fructose, while high fructose corn syrup is around 45% glucose and 55% fructose.

One of the reasons that added sugars are bad is that they can cause inflammation, which can lead to illness.

One study found that mice on high sucrose diets developed breast cancer that migrated to their lungs, which was caused in part by the inflammatory response to sugar.

Another 2011 study found that omega-3 fatty acid anti-inflammatory properties were diminished in mice on a high-sugar diet.

Furthermore, in a randomized clinical experiment in which participants drank normal soda, diet soda, milk, or water, only those who drank regular soda had higher levels of uric acid, which promotes inflammation and insulin resistance.

Sugar can also be dangerous since it contains an excess of fructose.

While little amounts of fructose are good in fruits and vegetables, ingesting high amounts of added sugars can be harmful to health.

Obesity, insulin resistance, diabetes, fatty liver disease, cancer, and chronic kidney disease have all been related to a high fructose diet.

Fructose also triggers inflammation among the endothelial cells that line your blood arteries, which is a risk factor for heart disease, according to studies.

In both rodents and humans, high fructose consumption has been demonstrated to enhance many inflammatory markers.

Candy, chocolate, soft drinks, cakes, cookies, doughnuts, sweet pastries, and certain cereals are rich in added sugar.

A diet heavy in sugar and high fructose corn syrup promotes inflammation, which can lead to illness. It may also have an anti-inflammatory impact like omega-3 fatty acids.

2. Deep-fried meals

Fried foods like French fries, mozzarella sticks, doughnuts, and egg rolls may cause inflammation in the body in addition to being heavy in fat and calories.

This is due to the fact that high-heat cooking methods, such as frying, can enhance the creation of hazardous substances such as advanced glycation end products (AGEs), which can induce inflammation and lead to chronic illness.

Frying can also increase the number of trans fats in cooking oils, which can contribute to inflammation.

According to certain studies, fried meals might alter the makeup of the gut microbiota, thereby increasing inflammatory levels.

Furthermore, several studies have revealed that eating fried foods may raise the chance of developing and dying from heart disease.

IN SUMMARY,

Foods that are fried can enhance the creation of toxic substances that might cause inflammation, such as AGEs and trans fats. Fried meals have also been related to an increase in the risk of chronic illness, according to research.

3. Carbohydrates that have been refined

Though carbs have had a poor name, many carbohydrate-rich foods are incredibly healthy and may be included in a well-balanced diet.

Excessive consumption of refined carbohydrates, on the other hand, might promote inflammation.

The majority of the fiber in refined carbohydrates has been eliminated. Fiber helps you feel full, improves blood sugar regulation, and feeds the good bacteria in your stomach.

Researchers believe that the refined carbohydrates in today's diet may promote the growth of inflammatory gut bacteria, increasing your risk of obesity and inflammatory bowel disease.

Refined carbohydrates have a higher glycemic index (GI) than raw carbohydrates. High-GI meals cause blood sugar levels to rise faster than low-GI foods.

In one study, children and adolescents with cystic fibrosis who followed a low GI diet for three months had substantial decreases in inflammatory markers when compared to a control group.

Another study found that a low GI diet might reduce levels of interleukin-6, an inflammatory marker, more efficiently than a high GI diet in persons with diabetes.

Candy, bread, pasta, pastries, certain cereals, cookies, cakes, sugary soft drinks, and any processed meals with added sugar or flour including refined carbs.

SUMMARY: High fiber, unprocessed carbohydrates are healthful; nevertheless, refined carbohydrates elevate blood sugar levels and cause inflammation, all of which may lead to illness.

4. Excessive alcohol consumption

Moderate alcohol drinking may be beneficial to one's health.

Higher levels, on the other hand, might cause serious difficulties.

In one 2010 research, participants who drank alcohol had higher levels of C-reactive protein (CRP), a sign of inflammation. CRP levels were greatest in those who drank more than two drinks each day.

People who consume a lot of alcohol may experience issues with bacterial toxins traveling out of the colon and into the body. This disorder, often known as "leaky gut," can cause extensive inflammation and organ damage.

To minimize alcohol-related health concerns, males should restrict their intake to two standard drinks per day and females to one.

IN SUMMARY,

Heavy alcohol use can cause inflammation and a "leaky gut," which spreads inflammation throughout your body.

5. Meats that have been cooked at high temperatures

Consuming high-temperature-cooked meats, such as bacon, sausage, ham, and smoked meat, has been linked to an increased risk of heart disease, diabetes, and some forms of cancer.

Grilling, barbecuing, roasting, frying, toasting, and searing are some more high-heat cooking methods.

High-temperature cooking causes the production of inflammatory chemicals known as AGEs.

AGEs are considered to contribute to chronic illnesses such as heart disease, cancer, metabolic syndrome, and type 2 diabetes, in addition to causing inflammation.

Interestingly, marinating meat in acidic solutions like lemon juice or vinegar before grilling or roasting will cut the number of AGEs in half.

Another technique to reduce AGE production is to cook meats for shorter periods and use moist heat cooking methods such as boiling, steaming, poaching, or stewing.

IN SUMMARY,

AGEs, which have been related to inflammation and chronic illness, are abundant in high-temperature-cooked meats, notably processed meats.

In conclusion

Inflammation can develop in reaction to a variety of causes, some of which are difficult to avoid, such as pollution, injury, or illness.

You do, however, have a lot more influence over things like your food.

To stay as healthy as possible, reduce inflammation by avoiding foods that cause it and consuming anti-inflammatory nutrients.

PART IV

Anti-Inflammatory Spices and Supplements

Inflammation is the body's natural response to injury or infection, and it frequently manifests itself as localized redness, swelling, discomfort, or heat. It may result in the loss of function of the tissues affected. Acute inflammation is often a limited and protective reaction to infection or damage. It is intended to help the body repair and restore normal tissue function.

Arthritis is characterized by joint inflammation, causing stiffness and edema.

Chronic inflammation occurs when inflammation lasts for an extended amount of time. Chronic inflammation can be caused by an infection, an autoimmune response, or an allergy.

Foods and spices that are anti-inflammatory

Anti-inflammatory foods have been identified. They may aid in the reduction of chronic inflammation and discomfort.

Anti-inflammatory benefits of omega-3 fatty acids present in fish, some nuts, and even chocolate have been recognized. The research on how efficiently these nutrients lower inflammation in the body is conflicting but encouraging. Spices are a simple method to integrate anti-inflammatories into your diet.

Ginger

Ginger is a spicy spice that is used in a variety of dishes. Most stores sell it powdered or as a raw root. Ginger has traditionally been used to alleviate stomach discomfort, headaches, and infections.

Ginger's anti-inflammatory effects have been hailed for years, and science has validated them.

Cinnamon

Cinnamon is a popular spice that is frequently used to flavor baked goods. But cinnamon is more than simply a tasty ingredient in our desserts. According to research, the spice possesses anti-inflammatory effects that help reduce swelling.

Keep a supply of cinnamon on hand and sprinkle some on top of your breakfast cereal and coffee.

Garlic

Garlic's anti-inflammatory qualities have been shown to alleviate arthritic symptoms. A little goes a long way. Fresh garlic may be used in practically any savory meal to enhance taste and health benefits.

If you don't like the taste, roast a head of garlic for a sweeter, milder flavor.

Cayenne

Cayenne and other spicy chili peppers have long been recognized for their health advantages. Capsaicinoids are natural chemicals found in all chili peppers. These are the anti-inflammatory qualities of spicy fruit.

Chili pepper is often regarded as a potent anti-inflammatory spice, so try a dash in your next recipe. It has long been used as a digestive aid, which is a bonus.

Black pepper

If cayenne is too spicy for you, you'll be relieved to know that the milder black pepper has also been linked to anti-inflammatory benefits. Black pepper, often known as the "King of Spices," has long been prized for its flavor as well as its antibacterial, antioxidant, and anti-inflammatory properties.

Black pepper chemical components, notably piperine, have been found in studies to be useful in the early acute inflammatory phase.

Clove

Cloves have been used as an expectorant and to alleviate stomach discomfort, nausea, and mouth and throat irritation. The research is still unclear, but it appears that they may have anti-inflammatory qualities.

Powdered clove complements baked items and some savory foods, such as robust soups and stews. Whole cloves can also be used to infuse flavor and nutrients into hot beverages such as tea or cider.

Anti-Inflammatory Supplements

Here are ten substances that have been shown in studies to help decrease inflammation.

1. Turmeric

Curcumin is a chemical found in turmeric, which is well-known in Indian cuisine for its vivid yellow color. It has several outstanding health advantages.

Curcumin, among other things, may help reduce inflammation in diabetes, heart disease, inflammatory bowel disease, and cancer.

It also appears to help with osteoarthritis and rheumatoid arthritis symptoms by lowering inflammation.

In one randomized controlled experiment, patients with metabolic syndrome who took curcumin had considerably lower levels of the inflammatory markers C-reactive protein (CRP) and malondialdehyde than those who took a placebo.

Another study found that when 80 persons with solid malignant tumors were given 150 mg of curcumin daily for 8 weeks, the majority of their inflammatory markers fell much more than those in the control group. Their quality of life scores improved dramatically as well.

While these advantages are feasible, curcumin is poorly absorbed into the bloodstream due to its low bioavailability (the rate at which your body absorbs a material).

2. Fatty fish oil

Omega-3 fatty acids, found in fish oil supplements, are essential for optimal health. They may aid in the reduction of inflammation linked with diabetes, heart disease, and other diseases.

The two main omega-3 fatty acids found in fish oil are eicosapentaenoic acid (EPA) and docosahexaenoic acid (DHA) (DHA). They are converted by your body to ALA, an important fatty acid.

DHA, in particular, has been found to have anti-inflammatory properties that lower cytokine levels and improve gut health. It may also reduce post-exercise inflammation and muscle damage, although additional study is needed.

According to certain research, DHA supplementation can considerably lower levels of inflammatory indicators when compared to a placebo.

Fish oil doses of less than 2 grams of EPA and DHA combined are safe; nevertheless, fish oil may produce fishy burps, foul breath, heartburn, or gastrointestinal discomfort. If you have a weakened immune system or are using a blood thinner, see your doctor before taking fish oil.

3. Ginseng

Ginger root is popular in cooking and has a long history of usage in herbal medicine. It's also used to alleviate indigestion and nausea, particularly morning sickness during pregnancy. Gingerol and zingerone, two components of ginger, may help decrease inflammation associated with a variety of health disorders, including type 2 diabetes. Ginger eating may also improve HbA1c (three-month blood sugar management) over time.

According to one study, giving persons with diabetes 1,600 mg of ginger daily for 12 weeks improved their blood sugar management and considerably reduced inflammation levels when compared to the control group.

Another research discovered that women with breast cancer who took ginger supplements had reduced levels of the inflammatory markers CRP and interleukin-6 (IL-6) compared to a placebo group, especially when paired with exercise.

Up to 2 grams of ginger per day is safe, but greater doses may cause blood thinning. If you're on a blood-thinning medication, consult your doctor before increasing your intake of ginger beyond what you'd normally use in cooking.

four. resveratrol

Resveratrol is an antioxidant present in grapes, blueberries, and other purple-skinned foods. Red wine, dark chocolate, and peanuts all contain it.

Its anti-inflammatory potential has been extensively researched in patients with chronic illnesses such as liver disease, obesity, and ulcerative colitis (UC), as well as in those who do not have chronic disorders.

In one trial, patients with UC (a kind of inflammatory bowel disease) were given 500 mg of resveratrol or a placebo everyday for 6 weeks. Quality of life, UC symptoms, and inflammation all improved in the resveratrol group.

Another study found that resveratrol supplementation reduced inflammatory markers, lipids, and blood sugar in obese adults.

Furthermore, an assessment of the benefits of resveratrol connected it to enhanced calorie expenditure and the potential to help decrease body fat. However, due to its low bioavailability, additional research is required.

The majority of resveratrol supplements include 150-500 mg per dosage and have no discernible negative effects. If you are on a blood thinner, you should consult with a doctor before using resveratrol.

4. Spirulina kind of algae.

Spirulina is a form of blue-green algae that has powerful antioxidant properties. It has been demonstrated in studies to decrease inflammation, promote healthy aging, and maybe boost the immune system.

Although most research has focused on the benefits of spirulina on animals, studies in older individuals have revealed that it may enhance inflammatory indicators, anemia, and immunological function.

Up to 8 grams of spirulina per day is safe, and because it comes in powder form, many people add it to shakes or smoothies.

There are no known serious negative effects, however, those with autoimmune disorders should avoid it since it has the potential to aggravate their illness due to its immune-strengthening qualities.

5. Vitamin D

Vitamin D is a fat-soluble substance that is crucial for immunological function and may have potent anti-inflammatory actions.

Researchers have discovered a relationship between low vitamin D levels and the prevalence of inflammation in multiple studies.

Researchers found that consuming 50,000 International Units (IU) of vitamin D every 20 days for four months reduced inflammation compared to a control group in a small, high-quality trial of 44 women with low vitamin D levels and premenstrual syndrome.

Similar outcomes have been observed in patients who are vitamin D deficient in addition to being obese.

Adults should not take more than 4,000 IU per day over the long term. Fat-soluble vitamins, including A, D, E, and K, are retained in fat cells and can accumulate over time, potentially causing toxicity.

6. Bromelain Enzyme.

Bromelain is a potent enzyme present in pineapple that contributes to the fruit's astringency. Bromelain is the reason why eating too much pineapple causes a burning feeling.

It does, however, have some anti-inflammatory qualities. Bromelain, in reality, has the same anti-inflammatory potential as nonsteroidal anti-inflammatory medicines (NSAIDs) but with fewer adverse effects.

Although little study has been conducted in humans on bromelain's anti-inflammatory qualities, it appears to be beneficial in lowering postoperative inflammation in persons following wisdom teeth removal.

The majority of bromelain pills include 500 mg per serving and have no recorded negative effects.

7. Green tea Extract

Green tea has long been used in traditional medicine because it contains chemicals that may give several health advantages, including epigallocatechin-3-gallate (EGCG), caffeine, and chlorogenic acid.

One possible advantage is that it is particularly anti-inflammatory.

In one small research of overweight males, 500 mg of green tea extract per day for 8 weeks, along with three times per week of exercise, significantly decreased inflammation compared to exercise alone or a placebo group that did not exercise.

Many of green tea's anti-inflammatory properties, according to researchers, are attributed to the EGCG it contains. As an antioxidant, EGCG can help reduce oxidative damage to your cells produced by free radicals, resulting in less inflammation.

You can purchase EGCG or green tea extract supplements, but keep in mind that green tea extract pills will include caffeine unless otherwise indicated. Green tea extract supplements are available on Amazon.

8. Garlic

Garlic, like ginger, pineapple, and fatty fish, is a well-known anti-inflammatory food.

Garlic contains a chemical called allicin, which is a powerful anti-inflammatory agent that may also help boost the immune system to better fight disease-causing microorganisms.

In one high-quality trial, 51 obese people were randomly assigned to receive 3.6 grams of aged garlic extract or a placebo every day for six weeks. The inflammatory indicators tumor necrosis factor-alpha (TNF-) and IL-6 improved significantly, according to the researchers.

They hypothesized that long-term aged garlic supplementation might help minimize the risk of chronic inflammation-related illnesses.

Garlic supplements are available in a range of doses, all of which are relatively safe and have few negative effects (except for garlic breath).

Furthermore, consuming just 2 grams of fresh garlic every day, or around one clove, may provide some anti-inflammatory effects.

9. Vitamin C

Vitamin C, like vitamin D, is a necessary vitamin that aids with immunity and inflammation. Because it is a strong antioxidant, it can help to decrease inflammation by neutralizing free radicals that cause oxidative damage to your cells.

It also helps to improve the immune system in a variety of different ways, which can aid in the regulation of inflammation, as inflammation is an immunological reaction.

Furthermore, high dosages are routinely administered intravenously to hospitalized patients suffering from severe respiratory infections such as influenza, pneumonia, and even COVID-19 to assist decrease inflammation.

Doses more than 2,000 mg, however, may cause diarrhea in healthy adults. Aside from that, vitamin C pills are relatively safe and symptom-free.

However, you may easily satisfy your vitamin C requirements by diet alone - green, red, orange, and yellow fruits and vegetables are all high in vitamin C.

In conclusion

Chronic inflammation may raise your chance of developing chronic diseases such as type 2 diabetes, heart disease, and autoimmune disorders.

Many supplements, which include anti-inflammatory minerals, antioxidants, or other chemicals, may aid in the reduction of inflammation in your body.

• Buy them from a reputable manufacturer, particularly one with a certified Good Manufacturing Practices (cGMP) facility (which assures they satisfy Food and Drug Administration criteria) that engages in third-party product testing.

• Stick to the dose recommendations on the product label.

• Consult your doctor first if you are pregnant or breastfeeding, have a medical condition or use medication.

Anti-inflammatory nutrients should ideally be obtained through whole meals, although supplements may be beneficial, especially if your diet is deficient in minerals and antioxidants.

PART V

Does Exercise Increase Immunity?

Could physical activity play a role in avoiding bacterial and viral illnesses and strengthening your immune system?

It turns out that regular physical activity might help you stay healthy and avoid ailments. Because exercise benefits your general health, it may assist support the operations of your immune system.

This article discusses the theories behind how exercise can help your immune system and if you should exercise when you're ill.

Is regular exercise beneficial to your immune system?

In a nutshell, sure. Exercise improves your body in a variety of ways, one of which is immune enhancement. However, there is one significant caveat: Workout frequency, length, and intensity are all important factors.

According to research, moderate-intensity exercise is the greatest way to enhance your immunity.

Exercise at a moderate to strong level for 60 minutes or less is generally recommended for the immune-boosting advantages of exercise. If you do this on a daily or near-daily basis, your immune and metabolic systems will continue to improve, building on earlier gains.

On the other hand, continuous high-intensity training, especially when not followed by adequate rest, might depress your immune system.

If you're a competitive athlete or training for an endurance event like a marathon, this is a crucial concern. In such circumstances, take extra precautions to provide your body with adequate recuperation time.

How much exercise would do?

Before we get into how physical activity might improve your immune system, it's necessary to talk about how much exercise you probably need for overall health.

Most individuals should engage in at least 150-300 minutes of moderate-intensity aerobic activity or 75 minutes of vigorous physical activity each week, according to the U.S. Department of Health and Human Services (HHS).

The HHS also suggests undertaking muscle-strengthening workouts involving all main muscle groups in your legs, hips, back, belly, chest, shoulders, and arms at least two days each week.

Being active on most days of the week is a great way to improve your overall health and well-being. It's also a good place to start if you want to improve your immune system.

What exactly is the Immune System?

We always hear about the significance of having a robust immune system, especially when it comes to preventing viruses, infections, and other disorders.

But what is the immune system precisely, and how important is it to your general health?

To begin, your immune system is made up of cells, organs, tissues, and even reflexes like the cough reflex. Its primary function is to resist or inhibit the spread of infections and other illnesses.

When your body senses an antigen — anything dangerous or alien, such as a virus, toxin, or bacterium — your immune system responds by destroying it in order to protect you. This is known as an immunological reaction.

During this response, your body produces antibodies that will aid in future defense against this antigen. Immunity is the defense your body is constructing.

The immune system is divided into two parts: the innate immune system and the acquired, or adaptive, immune system. The innate immune system is present at birth and activates immediately.

The innate system includes protection provided by mucous membranes and your skin, as well as the protection provided by immune system cells and proteins. It reacts to all bacteria in the same way.

As you mature, your body learns new things and acquires acquired immunity, which might come through a vaccination, exposure to a virus or disease, or antibodies from another person. If the innate system fails to eliminate the germs, acquired immunity might take control.

Because the acquired immune system remembers germs, it may particularly target the type of germ causing an infection and, ideally, keep you well.

IN SUMMARY,

The immune system consists of cells, tissues, and organs that work together to resist or restrict infections and other disorders.

Should you work out while you're sick?

If you're feeling under the weather, you might want to reconsider going for a run outside or to a crowded gym.

Exercising while ill may make you feel worse or postpone your recovery, especially if you have a temperature or are suffering from severe symptoms.

If your sickness is communicable, it also puts others at risk of being ill.

You'll need to make a list of your symptoms before deciding how to continue.

If you experience above-the-neck symptoms such as congestion, sneezing, sore throat, and runny nose, you may have a common cold and can engage in light to moderate activity.

However, if you have a fever or chills, body pains, a cough, or nausea, you may be suffering from a more serious illness, such as influenza or COVID-19.

If that's the case, missing your workout is generally a good idea.

IN SUMMARY, Before exercising while unwell, listen to your body and take note of your symptoms. If your symptoms are above the neck, you might be able to exercise. Rest is the greatest option if you have more serious symptoms, such as a temperature.

6 Ways Exercise Helps Your Immune System

A strong immune system defends your body from germs, viruses, and other pathogens that you come into contact with on a regular basis.

Here are six ways that exercise might benefit your immune system.

1. Exercise boosts cellular immunity.

A 2019 research review found that moderate-intensity exercise can boost cellular immunity by enhancing the circulation of immune cells in your body. By identifying an illness sooner, your body can better prepare for it in the future.

Aerobic exercise at a moderate to vigorous level for less than 60 minutes (an average of 30-45 minutes) increased the recruitment and circulation of the immune system's finest defense cells, according to the findings.

These findings suggest that regular exercise might boost immune defense activity by making you more resistant to infection and better prepared to cope with infectious pathogens that have already established themselves in your body.

2. Physical activity boosts body temperature.

Unless you're moving at a snail's speed, your body temperature will rise throughout most types of exercise and will remain raised for a short period after you finish.

What is the significance of this? It's widely assumed that this temporary boost in body temperature during and after exercise, similar to how a fever works, may prevent germs from developing and help your body better manage an illness. However, it is vital to emphasize that this assertion is not supported by evidence.

While this transient temperature increase is not as substantial as a fever, it may still be useful to your immune system.

3. Exercise improves your sleep.

Regular physical exercise can help improve the quantity and quality of sleep.

This is fantastic news because sleep deprivation may have a harmful impact on specific components of the immune system.

Some study suggests that those with a moderate quantity of sleep loss are at a higher risk of infection and the development of cardiovascular and metabolic problems due to a decrease in antibodies and the release of inflammatory cytokines.

4. Physical activity reduces the risk of heart disease, diabetes, and other disorders.

Exercise can lower cardiovascular risk factors, prevent or postpone type 2 diabetes development, boost HDL (good) cholesterol, and lower resting heart rate.

If you have one or more of these disorders, your immune system may struggle to fight infections and viral illnesses like COVID-19.

5. Exercise reduces stress and other illnesses including depression.

Working exercise after a hard day at work is popular for a reason: it reduces stress.

Moderate-intensity exercise, in particular, can reduce the production of stress hormones while also favorably impacting neurotransmitters in the brain that regulate mood and behavior.

Furthermore, regular exercise may provide a stress-reduction effect, which means that it helps you deal with stress with greater resilience and a better mood.

According to some studies, stress and depression can have a significant influence on the immune system's normal function, resulting in a low chronic inflammatory status that promotes infections, diseases, and other ailments.

6. Exercise helps to decrease inflammation

Inflammation is a natural immune system reaction used by your body to combat viruses or poisons.

Acute inflammation isn't always a concern, but when it goes unchecked, it can become chronic, possibly leading to a slew of inflammatory disorders.

Exercise has been demonstrated in studies to lower inflammation and keeps the immune system in balance — but the intensity of the exercise matters (21).

According to research, moderate-intensity exercise lowers inflammation, but high-intensity exercise might potentially increase inflammation (22).

What is the takeaway? Moderate exercise, along with adequate rest times, can boost the efficacy of your body's inflammatory immune response, decreasing your risk of chronic inflammation.

IN SUMMARY, Regular exercise can enhance your sleep, mood, stress levels, and the circulation of immune cells in your body, all of which contribute to a healthy immune system.

www.ingramcontent.com/pod-product-compliance
Lightning Source LLC
LaVergne TN
LVHW052105160826
845678LV00015B/3372

* 9 7 9 8 3 7 4 3 0 1 8 9 2 *